How to Tell if You Are Fat and What to Do About It

How to Tell if You Are Fat and What to Do About It

J.B. Whitaker, Ph.D.

Redwood Mountain Publishing

CONTENTS

DEDICATION vii

1 Introduction 1

2 Part 1: How to Tell if You Are Fat 4

3 Part 2: What to Do About It 12

4 Conclusion 21

First Printing: 2022

ISBN: 978-0-578-28008-0
eBook EISBN: 978-0-578-28066-0

Redwood Mountain Publishing
1060 E 200 S Unit 302
Brigham City, UT 84302

Visit the Redwood Mountain Publishing website using the QR code below or at www.redwood-mountainpublishing.com and subscribe to our mailing list to be notified of upcoming releases.

TO ALL OF US WHO STRUGGLE:
WE CAN DO HARD THINGS

Dr. J.B. Whitaker

I would like to give special thanks to Fred Rogers Productions for allowing me to use one of his quotes. His message has so much value for a community of people who struggle with weight loss and attach weight to worth. Mister Rogers was a master at acceptance, which is what many of us desperately need. I have no doubt he would have accepted me just as I am and that helps me to accept myself. I am grateful for his example.

1

Introduction

I do not know what percentage of humans struggle with weight loss. I am not a nutritionist who knows which of the hundreds of diet programs out there works best. I am not an exercise scientist who can tell you how much to work out and when. I am not a fitness guru who can lead you through an extreme body makeover. I am an economist. I currently weigh more than I ever have in my life. I contend with several formally diagnosed mental health issues. These are my qualifications for writing this book.

Why would anyone want to take diet and exercise advice from an overweight and depressed economist? That is a good question. All I can say is I desire to share a few lessons I have learned to help encourage others on their path to fitness, especially those of us who find ourselves, once again, at the beginning of this journey.

All of us go through periods of difficulty and find ourselves traveling down roads we could not have predicted and never wanted. Sometimes it is our own choices that lead us down a destructive path. Sometimes it is the choices of others that cause us harm. Some might argue that what we eat and how we exercise are within our control. That is true to an extent, but not entirely. Our socioeconomic circumstances and health, be it physical or mental, place restrictions on all of us. One can only choose what to eat if they have access to a variety of foods and the income to purchase them. One can only spend an hour at the gym if they can afford the gym or the hour. Someone who is allergic to certain foods is restricted. Someone who has arthritis may be limited in their mobility. Different people face different boundaries and some people's boundaries are more restrictive than others', but we have to acknowledge that legitimate boundaries to healthy eating and exercise do exist. However, within those boundaries, there is a degree of control each of us can achieve. What to eat? When to exercise?? Whether or not to improve our health???

As I stated, I currently weigh more than I ever have in my life. Over the last two years, I have struggled with depression, suicidal thoughts, anxiety, and a multitude of life changes that have affected me greatly. Giving up on life included giving up on a healthy diet and exercise regimen when I needed them most. This book is my attempt to take control and reintroduce healthy eating and exercise into my life because that is what I want for myself.

This is not a typical diet and exercise book. Rather than detail specific exercise routines or meal plans, I want you to change how you think about yourself, your diet, and your exercise regimen. By being aware of a few simple concepts, you will find yourself engaging in healthier living.

Before getting into the philosophical approach toward diet and exercise I propose, I provide some anecdotes I have journaled over the years that remind me I might be a little overweight. That's right. I keep a fat journal. In Part 1 below, I share these anecdotes and hope they make you laugh. They are all one hundred percent true events I experienced. Maybe you can relate through similar experiences of your own.

Some might call this humor self-deprecating, but it's only deprecating if being fat is bad or not okay. I don't subscribe to the premise that being fat is bad or not okay, so I don't consider these anecdotes to be self-deprecating. I discuss my philosophy on this in more detail in Part 2.

In Part 2 I also lay out what I think is the bare minimum that a person needs to do if they want to make a meaningful change to their diet and exercise routine. While the advice is directed toward those of us who struggle to motivate, the principles apply to everyone and even the fittest person might find some beneficial change to their perspective after reading them. I hope you find this book entertaining and motivating. Enjoy!

2

Part 1: How to Tell if You Are Fat

Over the last several years, I have had many experiences that give the impression I am a little heavy. I decided to start keeping a journal of these experiences. I present a few select anecdotes below. These are events I actually experienced, as strange and humorous as they may be.

Horse Horrors

I was going on a group horse ride and was assigned a horse that seemed a little smaller than the others. I mounted up and she snorted loudly, turned her head, and looked at me with huge, frightened brown eyes that seemed to say "are you kidding me?" The horse's legs began to quiver, slowly sinking into the mud below. The owner approached me and asked how much I weigh. I gave the honest answer and she said "you're going to need a bigger horse."

| 4 |

They searched for the biggest horse in the group. Her name was Sandy. About three minutes into the ride, I was at the very back of the group and Sandy was just pouring sweat down her neck and side. She was also voice breathing, similar to the noise I make when I stop to rest after getting up that first flight of stairs. The owner looked back from her mount and asked if I was okay. I pointed out that it was the horse making those noises and not me, which made her chuckle. Sandy and I made it through the ride. I dismounted and thanked her, but she just walked off without saying a word.

To Sit or Not to Sit

I keep track of how many chairs I have broken just by sitting in them. I am up to nine.

I was once in a wooden rocking chair when I heard the posts that attach the rocker to the seat crack. The entire left rocker buckled under. I wasn't even rocking!

I was sitting on a chair my father had inherited from his parents. It was a 1950's red vinyl chair with metal legs that were welded to the seat frame. I suddenly felt myself leaning to one side. I continued to sit there as the weld slowly gave way and the legs of the chair buckled under, sending me to the floor.

I was sitting in an office chair in front of my computer and leaning to one side on the armrest, which had been elevated to suit my height. I heard cracking and the entire armrest gave way, crashing down through its black, plastic casing, breaking it to pieces, and leaving the armrest detached and lying on the floor.

I was offered a small plastic chair at a work meeting. When I sat in it, the four legs slowly started to slide outward while the seat sank. The solution? They brought me three plastic chairs stacked on top of each other. That did the trick.

Three Amigos or Three Stooges?

I was sitting in a window seat waiting for a flight to finish boarding. Another large man was sitting in the aisle seat on my row. The middle seat had yet to be filled. I think we both saw him simultaneously, an even larger man than either of us walking down the aisle, searching for his seat. Sure enough, he was assigned the middle seat in our row. It was a full flight. There were no other options. No words were spoken during the flight.

Fats to Business Class Please!

I was looking for my seat when I saw it occupied by a rather large man. It was a middle seat on the front row. Before I could open my mouth, he acknowledged it was not his seat, but that his assigned seat was the window seat and he simply did not fit there. I was of course sympathetic and said I would take a crack at the window seat. I backed myself in and sat down, wedging myself between this man and the sloping interior wall of the plane. I do mean wedged. The man looked at me and said "I paid two hundred dollars to upgrade to that seat."

As we sat there looking uncomfortable, a flight attendant rushed by, stopped, backed up, and stared at us. She departed without a word and returned with two new seat assignments in business class, free of charge. That's right. I was upgraded to business class for being too fat. Nice!

Airplane Lavatories Are Not One-Size-Fits-All

While on an international flight I had to powder my nose. I entered the tiny lavatory and had difficulty turning around to close the door. The quick solution was to reach behind me to close and lock the door, which I did. It was then that I realized the type of nose powder I needed to use at the moment required me to be seated, not standing. I tried to turn around, but could not. I don't understand the physics of it, but I literally did not have enough space to turn around. I reached back up behind me, unlocked the door, and backed out into the aisle. I made eye contact with the people in line behind me as I silently turned around, backed myself into the lavatory, and closed the door.

Me? Water Ski?

I don't even want to talk about my water-skiing experience.

The Elevator Doth Protest

I was in an office building in Southeast Asia waiting for an elevator. There were two very petite women waiting with me. The elevator arrived and the women entered. I then stepped on, causing the elevator to make a long, loud buzzing sound, an alarm of sorts. The doors would not close. Confused, I stepped out of the elevator and the noise stopped immediately. I stepped back into the elevator and the buzzing started up again. The women began to giggle. I tried it one more time. Silence when I stepped off. Buzzing when I stepped on. I bid the laughing women farewell and took the stairs.

One at Bat and Two on Deck

I was eating a meal in a cafeteria when I had a moment of clarity. I was suddenly aware I had a fork with a piece of meat on it in one hand, a scoop of mashed potatoes on a spoon in the other hand, and joyfully chewed on a bite of something else. I remember feeling very excited for the next two bites and not being sure in what sequence I should consume them. The sudden realization that having a mouthful of food and two bites on deck simultaneously was not a civilized way to eat provided some evidence for the theory that "fat" is more a state of mind than a physical attribute.

Yog-Got to Be Kidding Me

I went to a yoga class at a swanky hotel in Southeast Asia. I entered the studio and took a mat. The small instructor looked at me, quietly walked over to the mat rack, grabbed a mat, and set it right next to mine. "You need two," he said matter-of-factly, the other patrons snickering as he walked back to the front of the studio.

How to Iron a Shirt Without an Iron

I was traveling for work and had not taken time to iron my shirt before I had to leave for an important meeting. I took the shirt directly from the suitcase and unfolded it. So many wrinkles! I could either be late or have a wrinkly shirt. I chose the latter. However, when I put the shirt on, the wrinkles somehow magically disappeared. It took me but a moment to realize why. Unfortunately, I found the experience quite satisfying, which has caused me to waiver much in my diet and exercise goals. If given the choice between being fat and having to iron, you might venture a guess as to where I stand.

The Most Sanitary Way to Open a Door

I was going to exit an office building that had a push bar handle. I wasn't fully conscious of it until I was out of the building, but I did not use my hands to open the door. I just walked straight through, my belly hitting the door handle and pushing the door open. With such doors, I now consciously no longer bother to use my hands. My belly gets there before I do and does all the pushing. It is a much more sanitary method for opening doors.

That Which Can Be Opened Cannot Be Closed

A car was parked in front of a house that had a grass strip between the sidewalk and the curb. I entered on the side of the car closest to the curb. The door opened without incident over the grassy portion, but after I sat down in the car, the bottom corner of the door dug into the grass as I tried to close it. It simply would not close with me in the seat. The harder I pulled on the door, the deeper it dug into the grass. Once I exited the car, the door once again closed just fine. I had to enter the car from the street side.

Leaning Into It

While I was carpooling to work, I shifted my position in the back seat from leaning right to leaning left. Everyone in the van grabbed on frantically to their seats, thinking we had been hit by another car. I explained to everyone there was no cause for panic; it was just me shifting my weight.

Fat Breathing

I was sitting on the couch when my daughter told me in an angry voice to "stop it!"

"Stop what?" I asked, genuinely confused.

"Stop breathing!" she said.

"Excuse me?" I replied, not understanding her demand.

"Stop your fat breathing. It's annoying."

It was at that moment I became aware of the phenomenon of fat breathing, but now I notice it everywhere. Many of us who are heavy have respiratory problems and if you are quiet and pay attention, you can hear how heavy our breathing is during meetings or in a waiting room. You can even hear it sometimes during those quiet moments in the movie theater.

Fat Breathing Confirmed

I was in the lobby of my apartment complex waiting for an elevator when the man next to me asked if I was okay and if I needed a doctor. He had heard my fat breathing and was genuinely concerned I might be having a medical emergency. I explained to him the phenomenon of fat breathing, for which he was grateful. The intervention of concerned citizens due to my fat breathing is a recurring event.

A Child's Prayer

My young daughter was offering our nightly family prayer when she prayed to the Lord in sincerity and faith that she would grow up to be big and fat just like daddy.

3

Part 2: What to Do About It

There are four main actions one can take to prime and prepare for any diet and exercise commitment:

- Accept yourself as you are now.
- Stop eating at the margin.
- Acknowledge why you eat.
- Just move!

Let's review these four actions and see if I can't convince you to adopt the corresponding truths for yourself.

Accept Yourself as You Are Now

I cannot stress enough how important it is to master this principle before starting on your diet and exercise journey. I know it seems counterintuitive. Some might logic that if you desire to change your physique, you must not be happy with your current physique or there is something wrong with how you are now. In fact, most exercise programs and practitioners use words like "improve" or "overcome." It is completely valid to set goals and work hard to achieve them, but that is not the most important consideration.

The premise that weight loss is good and weight gain is bad, or lean is good and fat is bad, is false. I concede being overweight can impact our health and limit our activities. This may be what people refer to as bad, but I still challenge that notion. It is neither good nor bad. It is simply "what is." There are many things out of our control that impact our health and limit our activities. Imagine someone with severe depression who takes medication that causes weight gain. Weight gain may affect their physical health and mobility, but given the nature of their circumstances, their boundaries, if you will, living with weight gain may give them their best life.

There are three possible outcomes to a weight-loss journey for someone who judges their worth based on weight or appearance.

1. They may lose weight and finally feel good about themselves.
2. They may lose weight, but fail to value their success, focusing instead on how much weight they still have to lose or some other physical flaw they identify.
3. They may not reach their weight loss goal, in which case the view of their self-worth becomes even more negative and severe.

By accepting ourselves as we are now, we eliminate the second and third outcomes as possibilities without sacrificing the ability to feel good about accomplishing a weight loss goal. If you learn to value yourself as you are now, the first outcome simply loses the word "finally" to become "they may lose weight and feel good about themselves."

I can say with confidence your self-worth and value as a human being is entirely independent of your weight, your physical appearance, your mental health, your mobility, your intellect, etc. You can love yourself as you are now *and* love yourself enough to not let yourself remain as you are now. To quote Fred Rogers: "Knowing that we can be loved exactly as we are gives us all the best opportunity for growing into the healthiest of people." In fact, Mister Rogers teaches the principle I'm trying to convey better than anyone else. If you want valuable weight loss motivation, go buy a book of Fred Rogers' quotes and you will understand why a successful diet and exercise journey can only start with accepting yourself as you are now.

Step one in starting a diet and exercise journey is accepting yourself as you are now.

> ## Truth #1: "I can accept myself as I am right now."

Stop Eating at the Margin

You find the words "at the margin" everywhere in economics. The marginal propensity to consume is the change in your consumption given a change in income. Diminishing marginal utility is the concept that the benefit you get from an additional unit of consumption diminishes with each unit consumed (that third bacon double cheeseburger at lunch is not as satisfying as the first one). There is a "marginal utility" principle at play when we are trying to diet and exercise and I believe it is the reason why many people fail with their diet goals. I'll try to explain the principle without using math.

For this example, let's assume that cheeseburgers are less healthy than salads. Consider a person who regularly eats a strict healthy diet. If you introduce one cheeseburger a month into their diet, what will be the magnitude of impact on that person's overall health? Not very large. Now consider the other extreme. Consider a person who regularly eats fast food. If you introduce a salad once a month into that diet, the overall impact on their health will be minimal. Here's the kicker though. If you were to add one cheeseburger each month to an already unhealthy diet, the overall health effects of that additional cheeseburger would also be negligible. I've used extreme examples, but regardless of a person's diet, each marginal bite of food has little impact on your overall health and that is true for every individual bite. The cheeseburger I eat today won't determine my overall health. It's what I eat over the course of a week, month, or year that will determine my overall health.

Why is it important to understand this concept? Because most of us make our daily consumption decisions at the margin. It won't hurt if I have this one bite. Just one piece of pie won't make a difference. When faced with a craving, whether we consciously stop to consider the impacts or proceed subconsciously, we recognize the consumption of this item at this moment won't have a big impact on our overall health. This allows us to continuously rationalize our food consumption.

So how do we stop eating at the margin? We consciously replace the economic truth with a more accurate physical truth: every bite counts. While it is true each cheeseburger taken individually may only marginally affect our overall health, it is also true each cheeseburger consumed adds calories to your calorie intake and expenditure equation. A marginal impact is still an impact. It counts. It contributes. It matters. That is true of everything you consume. So, make a conscious decision to stop eating at the margin. You might see how easily this principle would apply to an exercise regimen as well.

Most diets will tell you how much and what to eat. There are so many out there. You can pick one or not. Regardless, I encourage you to repeat to yourself the mantra of "every bite counts." If you accept this as truth, it will change what and/or how much you eat. You may still eat ice cream, but you'll do it knowing it counts. It contributes to your calories. It matters.

Truth #2: "Every bite counts."

Acknowledge Why You Eat

There are a variety of reasons why we eat, but how often do we take time to stop and analyze exactly why we are eating? Being mindful of why you eat can influence what and how much you eat. I came up with a few reasons why I eat:

- I am hungry.
- I am bored.
- I am depressed.
- I am celebrating something.
- I am on vacation.
- Something tastes really good, even if I'm not hungry.
- I am fueling a workout.
- I am recovering from a workout.

It is important to note I am only asking you to acknowledge why you eat. I am not suggesting that you should not eat when you are bored or depressed. I think all of the reasons I have listed are valid reasons to eat. It is learning to differentiate between your wants and needs. I may want six-pack abs, but when I am depressed, I really need that chocolate. On the other hand, some of my most satisfying months were when I was eating to fuel and recover from daily workouts.

Acknowledging why you are eating will give you a moment's pause to change your consumption choices if you so desire. If I acknowledge I'm only rummaging through the cupboards for something to eat because I am bored, I may intentionally decide to fill my time with something else. If it is because I am depressed, I may think of other coping mechanisms I have at my disposal. If I acknowledge I am not hungry, I may choose to save dessert for later or pass on it altogether.

I believe it is possible to simultaneously want and not want the same thing. This is particularly true with dieting and exercise routines. There are reasons we may want to exercise or eat healthy, which usually correspond with long-term goals, and reasons we want to skip a workout or break our diet, which usually correspond with short-term wants, but may also include short-term needs. Acknowledging why we are eating in each moment forces us to purposefully choose between short-term wants, long-term goals, and those rare but real moments of short-term needs.

Truth #3: "I can identify why I am eating."

Just Move!

In addition to changing our eating habits, we may also wish to change our daily exercise routine. The internet is full of excellent workout routines. Gyms abound. We have a lot of choices when it comes to working out. Remembering we all have our boundaries and we often exercise at the margin, I propose there are two things you can do to change your exercise routine from nonexistent to existent. The first is stretching and the second is walking. Doing one of these would meet the bare minimum requirement of an exercise routine and I find them to be the easiest starting points.

The beauty of stretching and walking is they are gateway exercises. If our boundaries permit, walking will turn into jogging or running. Stretching will turn into bodyweight exercises like pushups and sit-ups, which will, in turn, lead to weightlifting. Once we become loose and mobile and active, we may start craving sports or other more rigorous challenges. Or, we stay satisfied with walking and/or stretching and focus our energy and efforts on other priorities we may have. Either way is okay, but I will warn you, that once you start down the path of walking and stretching, you may find yourself craving the hard stuff more and more.

Don't fall into the trap of marginal thinking. If you are on a diet and exercise journey, then remember that thirty seconds of movement is better than zero seconds of movement. Some of my most satisfying exercise routines were when I was getting two to three hours of exercise a day. I would start with forty-five minutes of cardio in the morning. Then I would lift for an hour in the afternoons, followed by a sporting activity such as tennis, basketball, or boxing in the evenings. On some days I would even add teaching a spin class. This was a time in my life when I did not have responsibilities at home and when all of these activities were near where I lived and worked. I could not maintain such a schedule now and that is okay.

It might be worth a note of caution that it is possible for someone to exercise too much, though most of us don't struggle with such a problem. At some point, you will start to experience

JB

diminishing marginal utility from exercising. The fourth consecutive hour on the treadmill may be physically detrimental to your health. Depending on your circumstances, you may also be supplanting important aspects of your life with too much time at the gym, but this is a problem for future discussion.

I acknowledge that on some days, for some people, being able to stretch or walk may not *seem* to be possible. For example, those who suffer from severe depression find there may be days they cannot get out of bed. If that is your barrier, acknowledge it, but also acknowledge you can do some form of movement within the bounds of your reality. You can still stretch while lying in your bed. When that desire to just do something, anything, pushes through the clouds of depression, grab hold of it and take it for a walk.

I'll leave you with this final thought. I have never regretted exercising. No matter how sore I was or how difficult the task, I have never once regretted getting up and going.

Truth #4: "I can move."

4

Conclusion

I'll end this book with the diet and exercise routine that resulted in the most weight loss I have experienced in the shortest amount of time. First, I would start my day with a fasting cardio workout lasting forty-five minutes to an hour. Before breakfast, I would either walk briskly on an inclined treadmill or use an elliptical machine at high resistance, whatever got my heart rate up. I would stay hydrated, but I would not eat anything before I did my morning cardio. Afterward, I would eat healthy to recover, which was usually some sort of smoothie that included protein powder and a serving of fruit. During the day, I would eat to fuel my afternoon weightlifting. This included eating complex carbohydrates like brown rice, sweet potatoes, or oatmeal along with a healthy portion of protein like chicken, fish, pork, or beef. After I lifted weights, I would eat to recover, which included protein powder, vegetables like broccoli or asparagus, and another healthy portion of protein.

When you are committed to an exercise routine and eat purposefully to both fuel a workout and recover from one, the weight can drop safely and quickly.

I leave you with the following advice and truths.

- Accept yourself as you are now.
  - Truth #1: "I can accept myself as I am right now."
- Stop eating at the margin.
  - Truth #2: "Every bite counts."
- Acknowledge why you eat.
  - Truth #3: "I can identify why I am eating."
- Just move!
  - Truth #4: "I can move."

Remember, we all have boundaries that restrict us, but we are free to choose within those boundaries and often, with effort, we can move, or in some cases remove, those boundaries. I support you on your journey to living the life you choose and hope the principles I share in this book help you on your way.

www.ingramcontent.com/pod-product-compliance
Lightning Source LLC
Chambersburg PA
CBHW072158020426
42334CB00018B/2058